Mediterranean Diet

Mediterranean Diet Cookbook & Guide

Feel Great, Lose Weight, Gain Energy & A Healthy heart

Table of Contents

Introduction

All over the world, people are talking about the Mediterranean Diet, and many health professionals declare it to be the healthiest diet in the world, for people of all ages. It all began back in the mid 1980s, when statistics indicated that French people ate more saturated fats on average than Americans, British people, and many other nationalities. They also drank a lot of red wine and smoked a lot, yet they had a lower incidence of death from coronary heart disease (CHD). They also tended to be generally healthier, and live longer. The anomaly was dubbed the French Paradox.

This led researchers to wonder whether previous information that saturated fats contributed to CHD was flawed, but more studies in 1991 concluded that the reason the French were so healthy, despite drinking, smoking and eating more saturated fats than pretty much anyone else in the world was because of the rest of their diet. All of France eats in a similar way to the countries bordering the Mediterranean Sea, which means although they eat a lot of saturated fats, they also eat fish, which is high in Omega-3s for heart health, fruit and vegetables, which provide antioxidants, and the red wine. They also use a lot of olive oil, and eat few processed foods and fast foods, preferring to cook meals from scratch.

Statistics released in 1999 showed that 115 in every 100,000 American males aged between 35 and 74 died from CHD, but in France, that figure was a much healthier 83 in 100,000. So the researchers figured that the healthy diet mitigated the effects of smoking and even heavy drinking, and all of a sudden, the Mediterranean Diet was making headlines in all the health journals. And it's still big news today, because it gets results without excluding food groups, buying special foods and meal replacements, or sticking to ridiculously low calorie counts.

Actually the Mediterranean Diet is something of a misnomer, because it isn't a diet at all – it's a lifestyle eating plan. The word diet itself smacks of the temporary. People 'go on' and 'come off' diets, to fit into a bikini for their vacation, or to look good on the photos of a special occasion such as a wedding. Then more often than not, they regain the weight they'd lost, and maybe add a few more pounds for luck. So they become trapped in a yo-yo dieting cycle which messes around with their metabolism and makes it even more difficult to lose weight each time they 'go on a diet' in the future. Does that sound familiar? Then maybe it's time to try the Mediterranean Diet.

Countries that typically follow a Mediterranean-style eating plan include Italy, Spain and Greece – where the Mediterranean diet is said to have originated – Morocco, Portugal, Croatia and Cyprus. These days though, many countries are angling their cooking towards the Mediterranean style, with certain regional variations. That's because more people are catching on to the health and taste benefits of the Mediterranean Diet. And when you read how good it is, and feel how healthy you are after following it for just a short time, you will too!

Chapter 1:
The Basics of the Mediterranean Diet

Normally, the first chapter in a diet book deals with the rules, but as has been mentioned, this is not a diet, it's a lifestyle eating plan, so there are no rules, just basic guidelines you need to be familiar with if you are going to enjoy all the health and fitness benefits that the Mediterranean Diet has to offer.

There are no restricted foods, but if you need to lose weight as well as get healthy, you will need to control portions of high calorie foods, even the healthy ones such as nuts and olive oil. That's because to lose weight, you need to take in fewer calories than your body uses. You have to cut 3,500 calories to lose 1 lb of fat, so that means if you wanted to lose 1 lb a week, you'd need to reduce the operational calorie intake for your age and build by 500 calories a day. However, although the Mediterranean Diet is not a weight loss plan as such, if you follow the basics, you will naturally cut down on calories and may begin to lose a few pounds if you also factor in some extra exercise. These are the things you need to know to get started on the Mediterranean Diet.

Processed foods – cut them out or cut them down!

This is probably the single most important reason why the Mediterranean Diet is so healthy. Mediterranean mamas cook their food from scratch, and don't head to the grocery store for a microwave meal or send for a take out. Historically, these countries were poor, and people could not afford the foods enjoyed in some other cultures, or pay people to turn them into luxurious meals. They ate what they could grow, hunt or barter for, so fish, fruit and vegetables figured majorly in their diet, and the same is true today. Although they are more affluent these days, the culture of cooking from scratch is still deeply ingrained, and mothers teach daughters how to cook nutritiously and economically.

Yes, they eat cakes and desserts, but they're cooked at home, so there are no unhealthy trans fats or added salt, sugar and chemicals to improve the appearance and flavor and extend the shelf life. Trans fats and too much salt and sugar are responsible for several potentially serious chronic health conditions including cancer, CHD, diabetes and hypertension, and by cutting them down or cutting them out, you can do your health a big favor.

Choose healthy fats

Everyone needs some fat to stay healthy, but most people eat too much of the stuff. And all fat is not created equal – some fats are healthier than others. Olive oil is at the heart of the Mediterranean Diet, with extra virgin being preferred as it goes through less processing. Plant oils such as sunflower oil and rapeseed oil come next, but vegetable oils should be avoided.

Butter is better than margarine, but many Mediterranean countries only use a little butter in cooking – they don't spread it on bread, and that naturally cuts down on the saturated fat intake. Only the French consume a lot of butter – they eat it with bread, and use it for cooking and baking, and also in rich sauces.

Saturated fat – found in animal products – is automatically restricted on the Mediterranean Diet, as the people who follow it only tend to eat red meat occasionally. They prefer to get their protein from fish, poultry, rabbit and pulses and legumes such as chickpeas, lentils and beans, which figure largely in recipes.

Eat plenty of fish and seafood

As has been mentioned, many of the countries that follow the Mediterranean Diet surround the sea of the same name, or in the case of Portugal and parts of Spain, are located on the Atlantic coast. Therefore, there's a plentiful supply of fresh fish and seafood. Oily fish such as tuna, salmon, sardines, herring and mackerel is high in Omega-3 fatty acids, which are good for the heart and the immune system, lowering levels of harmful LDL cholesterol in the blood, and increasing 'good' HDL cholesterol. Fish is also low in calories and fat, so try to eat at least 2 – 3 servings a week.

Eat lots of fruit and vegetables

The Mediterranean region of Europe is like a giant market garden – you can grow every type of fruit and vegetable successfully in the long growing seasons that result from long hot summers and mild winters. The growers tend to produce food for local areas, so it is always in season, full of flavor, and ridiculously cheap. Because of this, the produce is not picked early and transported around the world in cold storage, so it's at the peak of freshness and vitamin content. Fruit and vegetables are high in antioxidants – especially brightly colored varieties such as carrots, peppers, broccoli, tomatoes, peaches, cantaloupe melons and citrus fruits.

Eat whole grains, pulses and legumes

Processed carbohydrates such as white bread, pasta and rice are unhealthy. They don't provide lasting filling power, which means your blood glucose levels are likely to be unstable, and they often contain extra sugar, salt and fats. Complex carbohydrates such as whole grain cereals, whole wheat bread and pasta and brown or wild rice are much better for you, and far more filling, which is exactly what you want if you're trying to lose weight.

Keep it simple

Mediterranean food is simple, wholesome and tasty. There are no rich sauces, and most of the recipes are derived from peasant food, so you will not get long lists of ingredients. That means cooking healthy, nutritious meals is easy – and much cheaper than buying convenience foods too. Herbs and spices are used for flavorings, rather than lots of salt, and the ingredients are always fresh and in season, so you get maximum flavor and vitamin content.

These are pretty much the basics of the Mediterranean Diet. As you can see, no foods are really forbidden, but you do need to be sensible about portion control if you are trying to lose weight. Otherwise, you can enjoy healthy, nutritious food from this moment. And if you're not sure how to go about cooking the Mediterranean way, the information and recipes in this book will soon get you started. We'll explain how to make the most of the foods available to you as part of this eating plan, and suggest ways to cook and serve them, giving you plenty of ideas for fantastic meals that will help you to stay healthy and make the most of life. Come on in – the food is lovely!

Chapter 2:
The Importance of Tomatoes in the Mediterranean Diet

Tomatoes are one of Nature's greatest gifts – they are low in fat and full of flavor, especially when they are grown in the sunny climate of the Mediterranean. They are also very versatile, whether you're serving them cold in a salad or salsa, or cooked in a sauce or recipe. Many Mediterranean recipes have tomatoes at their heart – think gazpacho, ratatouille, and pasta sauces, as well as bases for soups, stews and casseroles.

Here are some simple, multi-purpose ways with tomatoes, including some basic recipes where tomatoes are the star ingredients. Any tomatoes are suitable for these recipes, but large, beefy ones give the best yield and flavor.

Tomato paste recipe

It's not a very romantic name for something that's so full of flavor, but tomato paste is high on the list of favorites for Mediterranean meals. In its simplest form, it's one half of the breakfast dish tostada con tomate, as it's called in Spain. It's basically grated tomato, with added olive oil and pepper. It's also served with bread before lunch or the evening meal, or used to naturally thicken soups and stews.

- 2 -3 large tomatoes

- 10 – 15 ml olive oil (That's a dessert spoonful or a tablespoon)

- Freshly ground black pepper

- 1 – 2 cloves garlic, grated (optional)

Grate the tomatoes using a grater with an integrated bowl. To do this, cut the tomato in half, then rub gently over the grater surface. As you work, the skin will peel away to protect your fingertips. This method allows you to get every bit of flesh out of the tomato.

Now add the olive oil, pepper to taste, and garlic, if using. If you're serving the tomato paste for breakfast, it's best to omit this. Mix the ingredients together, and allow it to stand for at least an hour for the flavors to develop. Tomato paste will keep in a covered bowl in the fridge for 4 – 7 days. It can also be used as a spread on bread instead of butter. It works particularly well with cheese, ham, eggs and salad ingredients.

Tostada con tomate recipe

This is a popular breakfast in Spain and other Mediterranean countries, but it can be enjoyed as a snack at any time of the day or night. It's hearty and filling, yet healthy. It's a great opportunity to use up stale bread sticks, or you can just toast regular bread.

Now prick the bread surface with a cocktail stick or a fork, and drizzle a little olive oil over it. Then spoon over a generous serving of the tomato paste, and season to taste with extra pepper, and a little salt if required. That's it – enjoy!

Gazpacho recipe

Gazpacho is a traditional cold soup, usually served in Spain, but variations of it are also served in other countries, under slightly different names. The name is thought to originate from the Latin word for 'crumbs.' The soup has very few ingredients, and the tomatoes are the stars. Serve as a starter to a meal, or a healthy, anytime snack.

This recipe for a traditional gazpacho serves 4 – 6 people:

Ingredients

- 5 slices stale white bread (or a section of stale bread stick)

- 900 g ripe tomatoes

- 2 garlic cloves, crushed

- 5 tbsps extra virgin olive oil

- 2 tbsps lemon juice, lime juice or wine vinegar

- 120 ml ice cold water

- 1 tsp salt

- Large pinch of paprika – for a different flavor, try smoked paprika

Garnishes

- 2 slices of bread, shallow fried in olive oil and cut into croutons

- 1 hard-boiled egg, chopped

- 1 small red onion, chopped

- ½ red pepper and ½ green pepper, finely chopped

- 3" piece of cucumber, finely chopped

Soak the bread in cold water for 15 – 20 minutes, then press out the water from the bread in a sieve and blend it with the garlic until smooth. De-seed and chop the tomatoes. Blend all the ingredients together before adding the salt and paprika. Drizzle in the olive oil, followed by the lemon juice or vinegar. Keep the blender running all the time. Add the water, using a little more or less to obtain the consistency you want. If you want the gazpacho to be really smooth, whizz it in a food processor, but it's nice to have some texture, and it's more filling that way.

Chill the gazpacho until you are ready to dish up. Serve the garnishes separately so that everyone can help themselves.

Tomato frito (puree) recipe

Tomato frito is the Mediterranean version of tomato puree, and like most things Mediterranean, it's usually home made from fresh ingredients, for use as the base for sauces, soups, stews and casseroles. It also makes a great fresh, additive free tomato sauce for hamburgers and bacon sandwiches.

You can buy ready-made tomato puree in cartons or jars, but once you've made your own and seen what a fresh taste home-made tomato frito imparts to your cooking, you'll never want to go back to bought sauces. The basic recipe is so simple; it's not even a recipe really.

Peel at least two large, ripe tomatoes and chop them. The easiest way to do that is using a potato peeler. Then chop the tomatoes, heat the olive oil and fry the tomatoes, adding a pinch of salt for each couple of tomatoes you use. Fry the tomatoes for 15 minutes or so, until they are the consistency of a thick sauce. If you have a glut of tomatoes, you can use a large pan and cook them in bulk. They will keep in the fridge in a covered, non-metallic bowl for up to a week.

As you can see, tomatoes are an important component of the Mediterranean Diet. They can be enjoyed raw or cooked, and indeed, cooked tomatoes are believed to be higher in antioxidants than raw tomatoes. They also impart a lovely fresh flavor to any dish they are incorporated into.

Chapter 3:
Soups and stews

Many cultures have soups and stews at the heart of their diet, and the Mediterranean countries are no exception. With vegetables being plentiful and economically priced, and stews and soups being healthy, economical and filling, they are a popular choice in the Mediterranean region. Often they feature herbs and paprika, and even bacon lardons, for flavor. Many soups and stews have a tomato base, with either tomato paste or cooked tomato frito among the ingredients, so they're low in fat and calories. Here are some great Mediterranean inspired soups and stews.

Lentil, bacon and sweet potato soup recipe

This is a good standby soup when the store cupboard is running low, and you want something hearty and filling. The sweet potatoes break up in the soup and impart a lovely color and flavor, as well as helping to thicken it. These recipes used cooked lentils and other pulses, which are available in jars or cans, but for more economy you can use the dried equivalent. Just remember to soak them for the required time before beginning to cook. The quantities below provide 4 large servings, or you can make a larger amount and freeze it for another day.

Ingredients

- 150 – 200 gms smoked bacon lardons

- 1 large or 2 small leeks

- 2 large carrots

- 1 large or 2 medium sweet potatoes

- 1 large green pepper

- 1 small can sweet corn or garden peas

- 1 x 540 g jar of cooked lentils, drained and rinsed

- I standard tin of whole tomatoes

- Sea salt and ground black pepper to taste

- Fresh or freeze dried parsley

- 1 bay leaf

- Olive oil

- 2 vegetable stock cubes

- Approx. 1 liter of water

Wash and chop the leeks, or cut them into rings. Peel the carrots and sweet potatoes and cut into 1" chunks. Deseed the pepper and chop.

Heat a little olive oil and soften the leeks, then add the bacon lardons, carrots, sweet potatoes and pepper. Cook for a few minutes until the vegetables begin to soften.

Add the lentils, tomatoes, seasonings, stock cubes and water, give it a good stir, then turn the heat down and simmer for at least one hour, stirring occasionally. The soup is ready when it has thickened, but there are still small chunks of sweet potato in it. At this point, stir in the sweet corn or peas and cook for a few more minutes. Serve with crusty bread.

Roasted red vegetable soup recipe

This particular soup has an outstanding flavor, with its combination of roasted red peppers, carrots, aubergines and onions and raw grated tomatoes, and it's so quick and easy to make.

The soup is smooth, so for added texture and color, add a topping before serving. Use croutons, or dry fry smoked bacon lardons until crisp then top the soup with these. Another great topping of mine is diced green and yellow peppers. Grated raw carrot makes another colorful, crunchy topping. Maybe you can come up with your own toppings, given a little thought.

Ingredients for 4 – 6 servings

- 4 large red peppers

- 4 large carrots

- 2 aubergines

- 2 red onions

- 6 – 8 large ripe tomatoes

- 3 – 6 large cloves of garlic, depending on your taste

- 6 tbsps olive oil

- 2 teaspoons of paprika

- Sea salt, freshly ground black pepper and ground chili flakes

- Around a liter of vegetable or chicken stock

- Chopped fresh parsley or freeze dried parsley to garnish

Cut stalks from peppers, halve and scrape out ribs and seeds. Scrub the carrots, halve them down the middle, then cut them into chunks. Cut the tops from the aubergines, and then halve and quarter them lengthwise. Peel the onions and cut them into 8 to 10 wedges, depending on their size. Peel the garlic cloves and leave them whole.

Add oil to one or two large roasting pans, then toss vegetables. The pans should be large enough for the vegetables to be spread out in a single layer. Season them with salt, pepper and chili flakes and roast them at 200 degrees C for 30 minutes or so. The vegetables should be soft and slightly charred at the edges but not burned black.

While the vegetables are cooking, grate the tomatoes and combine them with the paprika.

Once the vegetables are cooked, blend them until smooth in several batches, adding a little stock each time. Transfer the blended stock and vegetables to a large saucepan and heat it gently. Add extra stock if necessary to obtain your preferred consistency. Don't allow the soup to come to the boil, since this could impair the flavor.

Add extra seasoning if it's needed, sprinkle the soup with fresh or freeze dried parsley and add the topping of your choice. Serve with fresh crusty bread.

Chunky fish soup recipe

This is a nice hearty fish soup that is brimming with Mediterranean ingredients. It makes a delicious low fat lunch or supper, or a super starter. For extra color, substitute the sweet corn with diced red and green peppers, added to the pan with the leeks. If you like a little spice in your soup, add some paprika and a chopped fresh chili. Ring the changes by adding fresh or dried pasta shapes instead of potatoes. This really is a versatile recipe that you can tailor to individual tastes.

Ingredients for 4 – 6 servings

- 2 tbsp olive oil

- 2 leeks, finely sliced

- 550g potatoes, cubed

- 1 liter of fish stock, from a cube or freshly made

- Zest of 1 lemon

- 300ml semi skimmed milk

- 330g can sweet corn, drained

- 250g fresh or frozen salmon or tuna, cut into chunks

- 250g fresh or frozen white fish, cut into chunks

- Fresh or freeze dried parsley to garnish

- 2tablespoons of Greek yogurt (optional)

- Salt and pepper to taste

Heat the oil and add the leeks to pan, cooking until softened. Add the potatoes and cook for 5 minutes. Add the stock, lemon zest, salt and freshly ground black pepper and cook for another 15 minutes. Then remove around half of the vegetables and set aside.

Put the remaining soup mixture into a blender with the milk and liquidize until it's smooth. Return it to the pan and add the sweet corn, fish and reserved vegetables. Cover the pan and heat the soup through for around 5 minutes until the fish is just cooked. Don't allow the mixture to boil, as it will destroy the delicate flavor of the soup and make the fish tough.

Stir in the parsley and the yogurt, and season the soup to taste. Serve with fresh crusty bread or croutons.

Chickpea and potato stew recipe

This tasty stew of Spanish origin is quick, easy and economical to prepare, and since you get a good protein hit from the chickpeas, you don't need any meat with it. The flavor stands up for itself. Before you get going, here's a tip for preparation. The thick gravy and unique flavor of this stew is down to extra starch being released from the potatoes. When you've peeled them ready for slicing, cut the slices halfway through, and then just break them away from the main potato. That's because uneven surfaces allow the potato to release more starches into the cooking liquid than straight cuts.

Grating tomato is a Spanish culinary technique that ensures that there are no irritating slivers of skin in the finished dish. It also helps to thicken the sauce and enhance the flavor, so don't even think of chopping the tomato to save time. Hints on grating tomatoes safely are covered in the previous chapter.

Ingredients for 4 servings

- 4 medium potatoes plus 1 small one

- 1 large ripe tomato

- 1 large onion, chopped

- 1 – 2 cloves garlic

- 1 x 540g jar of cooked chickpeas (garbanzos), drained and rinsed

- Olive oil

- Small knob of butter

- Sea salt and freshly ground black pepper

- 1 tablespoon of fresh or freeze dried parsley

- A little fresh or dried thyme

- 2 level teaspoons of paprika – smoked paprika gives a very different flavor. Try both, and see which you prefer.

- Small glass of red wine (optional)

- 1 tbsp tomato puree or tomato frito

- Optional extra vegetables: anything you fancy or have available from the following: red or green peppers, courgettes, celery, green beans. Aubergines don't work well with this recipe.

Heat some olive oil to soften the onions and garlic. Then add a small knob of butter and the red wine, if you wish. Add the parsley, thyme, salt and pepper.

Grate the tomato directly into the pan, then add the paprika and some water to prevent the mixture burning. Cook everything for a few minutes.

When you're ready, add the chickpeas and large sliced potatoes, tomato puree, any optional vegetables and enough water to cover everything in the pad. Simmer for around 45 minutes, then grate the small potato directly into the stew to help thicken the sauce. Cook the stew for at least another half hour, until everything is cooked through and the sauce is really thick.

Serve it with fresh crusty bread. This stew is even better if you cook it the day before you need it, since this gives the flavors lots of time to develop and combine together.

For a differently flavored dish, or if you prefer your stews to have at least some meat, try adding some smoked bacon lardons with the onions and garlic. Or add meatballs or sliced chorizo sausage at the same point. Experiment until you find the version you really like.

Recipe for ratatouille

Ratatouille is a typically Mediterranean dish. It's packed with fresh flavors, and even fresher vegetables. It can be served as a side dish to a meal of pan fried chicken breasts, or as the main course of a vegetarian meal, accompanied by a jacket baked potato, fresh wholemea bread, wild rice or whole wheat pasta.

Ingredients for 4 servings

- 500g of large ripe tomatoes

- 1 medium red onion, chopped pr sliced

- 1 -2 cloves of garlic, crushed

- 1 large courgette, cut into 1" wedges

- 1 green pepper, roughly chopped

- 1 red or yellow pepper, roughly chopped

- 1 small – medium aubergine, cut into 1" wedges

- 2medium carrots, roughly chopped

- Salt and pepper to taste

- A glass of red wine (optional)

- Fresh or freeze dried parsley

- 500 mls chicken or vegetable stock

- Olive oil

Heat the olive in a large pan, then soften the onions and garlic. Add the rest of the vegetables and sauté lightly, until the vegetables are browed and sealed. Now add the tomatoes, seasoning, red wine and stock. Bring to the boil and then turn down and allow to a simmer for 45 minutes – one hour. Serve with the accompaniments of your choice.

Pisto recipe

Pisto is something that doesn't crop up much in Spanish cuisine - a vegetarian dish. It's basically the Spanish equivalent of French Ratatouille, and it can be enjoyed as a main course its own, or served up with chicken, sausages, fish, pasta, eggs – or pretty much anything else you can think of! It's also a dish that can be eaten hot or cold, so it is a versatile addition to your recipe collection.

Ingredients to serve 4

- 50 mls of olive oil

- 1 large onion, chopped

- 1 red or green pepper, chopped

- 2 cloves of garlic, chopped finely

- 1 large aubergine, chopped into chunks

- 1 can of whole tomatoes

- 1 large courgette, sliced

- Fresh or freeze dried parsley – as much or as little as you like.

- Salt and ground black pepper to season

Prepare the vegetables. Make them as fine or as chunky as you like, as long as they are in more or less uniform pieces. Heat the oil in a large pan and add the onions, peppers and garlic. Fry until they soften, and then add the aubergine, and fry for a few more minutes. Finally, add the courgettes, tomatoes and seasoning, cover and cook for around 15 minutes. Try not to overcook this dish, because you really want the vegetables to retain their texture and color. That's all there is to it! Simply serve the pisto with fresh crusty bread for a really tasty treat.

You can also add smoked bacon pieces to ring the changes. Reduce the amount of oil, and fry the lardons for a couple of minutes before adding the onions, peppers and garlic. For a somewhat different accompaniment, toast slices of bread, then sprinkle with grated cheese and brown under the grill. The crispness of the toast contrasts nicely with the Pisto, while the cheese adds another flavor and makes a filling meal for vegetarians.

Pisto is a versatile dish that is quick and easy to prepare. It's also a great way of aiming towards your 5 portions of fruit and vegetables a day. Enjoy!

Mixed bean with morcilla stew recipe

Mixed bean stew with morcilla is light enough to eat in the summer if you fancy a change from barbecues and salads, even though it's a stew. This is a tasty version of the Andalucian classic.

Morcilla is a black sausage made with blood, similar black pudding from England. Don't let the look of the sausage put you off; the flavor is great and a little goes a long way. Use jars of cooked beans if you don't want to spend time soaking dried beans. The flavor is a little different, but it is pretty much impossible to say whether one is superior to the other.

Prepare the tomatoes and potatoes using the same technique described in the chickpea and potato stew recipe. It freezes well, so the recipe is made with complete jars of beans.

However, if you want to make less stew, here is a delicious way to use up the rest of the beans. Sweat a large onion and a clove of garlic in some olive oil. Add a large grated tomato, a tablespoon of tomato puree, salt, pepper, some grated chili flakes and the drained and rinsed beans. Heat through and serve with chorizo sausages or slices of lomo (cured pork) and crusty bread.

Ingredients (for 8 servings)

- 1 jar each of cooked chickpeas, white beans and lentils, drained and rinsed.

- 300 - 400g morcilla, chopped into ½" pieces.

- 3 – 4 large potatoes peeled and roughly sliced.

- 1 – 2 tbsps olive oil

- 1 large onion, chopped

- 1 green or red pepper, chopped

- 2 -3 cloves garlic, chopped

- 1 large or 2 medium ripe tomatoes, grated

- 2 tbsps tomato puree

- 500mls chicken stock from a cube

- Sea salt, freshly ground black pepper

- 1 tsp paprika

- ½ tsp ground chili flakes, or a small fresh chili, chopped

- 1 glass red wine (optional)

- Freeze dried parsley to garnish

Heat the oil in a large pan and soften the onion and the garlic. Add the peppers, tomato and tomato puree and cook for a few minutes.

Add the rest of the ingredients except for the morcilla and bring the stew to the boil. You may need some extra stock or water to cover everything. Simmer for around an hour, and then add morcilla. Cook for a further 20 – 30 minutes. The morcilla will break up and thicken the stew, but if you would like some chunks of morcilla in the stew, cut it into 1" cubes rather than ½".

Allow the stew to stand for a few minutes before serving to allow all the flavors to combine. Better yet, make stew the day before you're going to eat it. Garnish with the parsley and serve with fresh crusty bread.

Use these recipes to get you started on the Mediterranean way of cooking. They introduce you to some of the basic cooking techniques used in the region, and also the staple ingredients you will need to keep on hand. Remember to use lots of vegetables, and flavor your food with herbs and spices rather than using too much salt.

Why not experiment and grow your own herbs? Parsley, basil, oregano, thyme and rosemary are all commonly used in Mediterranean style recipes, and if you grow your own, you will have a never-ending supply of fresh herbs. They impart a very different flavor to dried herbs, but if you can't manage to get fresh herbs or grow your own, freeze dried herbs are a good alternative. Now let's take a look at some great ways with meat, poultry and game.

Sweet and sour Sicilian rabbit stew

This dish is all about creating magic with lean rabbit, capers, olives and loads of vegetables. The honey reduction and the red wine vinegar are responsible for the sweet and sour flavors to this dish.

This recipe for rabbit stew serves 12 people.

Ingredients:

- 1 teaspoon of sea salt, divided
- 2 tablespoons of honey
- 2 fresh rabbits, cut into 12 pieces
- ½ cup of extra virgin olive oil, divided
- 1 cup of dry white wine
- 2 cups of finely diced red onions
- ½ teaspoon of freshly ground black pepper
- 3 cups of peeled and diced potatoes
- 2 cups of diced carrots
- 3 pounds of small cherry tomatoes, cut in halves
- 2 cups of finely diced celery
- ½ cup of capers, rinsed well
- ½ cup of pine nuts

- 1 cup of green olives, pits removed and coarsely chopped

- ½ cup of red wine vinegar

Take the rabbit pieces first. Season them well with ½ teaspoon of salt and pepper. Allow it to rest. As the seasoned rabbit pieces are resting, take a large pot and place it over medium heat. Add around 4 tablespoons of olive oil to it and heat it. Add the rabbit pieces to the pot and cook them for around 4 to 8 minutes, turning them a couple of times. This should be sufficient time for the rabbit to turn golden brown in color. Transfer the cooked rabbit to a shallow bowl.

Now, pour the white wine into the pot. Increase the heat to medium high. Cook the wine for around 2 minutes. This should be sufficient time for the wine to get reduced. Now, pour the reduced wine into the bowl, over the rabbit pieces. Cover the bowl with a lid. This will keep the rabbit warm.

Add the remaining olive oil to the pot and heat it over medium heat. Add the diced onions to the pot and cook for around 2 to 3 minutes. This should be sufficient time for the onions to soften. Now, add the celery, carrots and potatoes to the pot and cook for another 5 to 6 minutes. This should be sufficient time for the vegetables to get cooked and turn soft. Finally, add the olives, tomatoes, pine nuts, tomatoes and capers to the pot and stir well. Cook the mixture for another five minutes. This should be sufficient time for the tomatoes to break down.

Add the rabbit pieces and wine to the pot and mix well. Cover the pot with a lid and cook the mixture at medium low heat for around 35 minutes.

As the rabbit is getting cooked, take a small saucepan. Add the red wine vinegar and honey to it and whisk well. Place the pan over high heat and bring the mixture to a boil. As the mixture starts boiling, reduce the heat to medium low and let it simmer for around five to eight minutes. The mixture should get reduced to half in this time.

At the end of 35 minutes, add the vinegar mixture to the pot and stir well. Now, increase the heat to medium and cook the mixture, uncovered, for an additional ten minutes. Add the remaining salt to the mixture and stir well.

Serve the stew hot.

Hunter's chicken stew

This Italian dish is loaded with the richness of tomatoes, mushrooms and onions. It is the perfect accompaniment for egg noodles.

This recipe of chicken stew serves 16 people.

Ingredients:

- 6 medium onions, peeled and chopped finely

- 4 teaspoons plus 4 tablespoons of extra virgin olive oil, divided

- 1 cup of all-purpose flour

- 12 cups of cold water

- 4 cloves of garlic, finely minced

- 4 teaspoons of salt, divided

- ½ teaspoon of freshly ground black pepper, plus more to taste

- 24 bone-in chicken thighs, skinless and trimmed

- 3 pounds of button mushrooms, cut in halves

- 8 plum tomatoes, finely chopped

- 2 cups of dry white wine

- 4 bay leaves

- 2 cups of reduced sodium chicken broth

- 2 2/3 cups of cornmeal

- 4 teaspoons of finely chopped fresh rosemary

- 2 tablespoons of finely sliced fresh basil

Place a large Dutch oven over a medium low heat. Add 4 teaspoons of the olive oil to it and heat it. Next, add the chopped onions to it and cook it for around 5 minutes, stirring occasionally. Add in the minced garlic next and cook for around 2 to 4 minutes. This should be sufficient time for the onions to turn soft and translucent. With the help of a slotted spoon, transfer the cooked onions to a bowl and keep it aside. Now, remove the pot from the heat.

Take a shallow dish and add the flour to it. Season the chicken pieces well with 1 teaspoon of salt and pepper. Now, dredge the seasoned chicken thighs in the flour. To discard any excess flour, shake the pieces gently.

Now, return the Dutch oven to the stove. Add one tablespoon of oil to it and add six thighs to it. Cook it over medium high heat for around 2 to 4 minutes per side. This should be sufficient time for the chicken thighs to get browned well. Repeat this step with the remaining chicken thighs. Transfer the cooked pieces to a plate.

Now, pour the white wine into the pot and cook for around one minute. Ensure that you scrap off any browned chunks of chicken with a wooden spoon. Add the mushrooms, chicken broth, tomatoes, rosemary and bay leaves to the pot and stir well. Add the cooked onions to the pot at this stage. Add the cooked chicken pieces to the pot next. Let the mixture simmer. Cover the pot with a lid partially and cook the mixture for around one hour, stirring occasionally. This should be sufficient time for the chicken to turn tender.

As the chicken mixture is getting cooked, take a large saucepan. Add the cornmeal, salt and water to it and combine well. Allow the mixture to boil, while stirring continuously. Let the mixture boil till it thickens. This should be done in around 5 minutes. Now, add the cornmeal mixture to the stew and reduce the heat to low. Allow the mixture to simmer for around 45 minutes to an hour. This should be sufficient time for the mixture to turn thick and creamy.

Once the chicken mixture is cooked, transfer the chicken pieces to a plate and cover it with foil to retain its warmth. Increase the heat to medium high and allow the liquid in the pot to boil for around 10 to 15 minutes. This should allow the liquid to thicken. Season the liquid with the remaining pepper and salt and mix well. Return the chicken pieces to the pot. Discard the bay leaves before transferring the chicken to serving plates. Garnish with basil and serve hot.

Moroccan chorba

This Moroccan soup is packed with nutritious and flavorsome vegetables, chunks of meat and pasta. This vibrant colored soup owes its color to the addition of turmeric.

This recipe for Moroccan chorba serves 12 people.

Ingredients:

- 2 medium onions, peeled and finely diced

- 4 tablespoons of extra virgin olive oil

- 4 teaspoons of ground turmeric

- 12 cups of reduced sodium beef broth

- 2 pound of beef stew meat, trimmed and chopped into cubes of ½ inch thickness

- 2 14-ounce cans of diced tomatoes

- 4 carrots, peeled and finely diced

- 4 ounces of whole wheat angel hair pasta, cut into smaller pieces

- 4 stalks of celery, sliced thinly (leaves included)

- 4 small turnips, peeled and finely diced

- Pinch of saffron threads

- 16 sprigs of fresh cilantro, plus some more for garnish

- 24 sprigs of flat leaf parsley, plus some more for garnish

- 2 large zucchinis, peeled and diced finely

- 1 teaspoon of freshly ground black pepper

- 2 to 4 teaspoons of salt

Take a Dutch oven and place it over medium high heat. Add the chopped onions and turmeric to it. Stir well to ensure that the onions get coated well with the turmeric. Add the beef to the pot and cook for around 4 to 5 minutes, while stirring occasionally. This should be sufficient time for the onions to get cooked and turn tender. Now, pour in the beef broth and stir well. Add the chopped turnips, tomatoes (along with their juice), carrots, saffron and celery to the mixture and mix well. Use a kitchen string to secure parsley sprigs and cilantro sprigs. Lower the string into the pot and let it cook with the other ingredients in the pot. Bring the mixture to a boil. Once the soup starts boiling, cover the pot with a lid and reduce the heat. Let it simmer for around 45 to 50 minutes. This should be sufficient time for the meat to get cooked and turn tender.

Once the meat has turned tender, add the zucchini to the pot and cook it, with the lid on, for around 8 to 10 minutes. This should be sufficient time for the zucchini to turn soft. Add the pasta to the pot next and cook for around 4 to 10 minutes. The cooking time entirely depends on the type of pasta. This should be sufficient time for the pasta to get cooked and soft. Remove the parsley and cilantro sprigs now. Season the soup with salt and pepper. Make sure that you don't add too much salt, since the broth will already have some salt in it.

Remove the soup from the heat and transfer it to serving bowls. Garnish it with parsley and cilantro leaves and serve hot.

Chapter 4:
Meat, Poultry and Rabbit

In the Mediterranean region and the Mediterranean Diet, chicken, poultry, fish, seafood and rabbit are eaten much more frequently than red meats such as beef and lamb. Pork is also classed as a red meat, and when this is eaten, they tend to eat lean cuts such as tenderloin rather than fatty belly pork. This means saturated fat is naturally restricted, and most of the visible fat is removed before cooking too.

Meat and poultry tends to be either pan fried or served in a casserole rather than roasted while rabbit is usually served in stews and casseroles, or rice dishes such as paella. Here are some recipes to help you with cooking meat, poultry and rabbit the Mediterranean way

Paprika chicken recipe

Paprika is a commonly used spice in Mediterranean cooking. It gives food flavor without the spicy heat of Mexican or Indian food. Smoked paprika gives a slightly different flavor to the regular stuff, and if you want to add thickening as well as flavor to stews and casseroles, mix together some corn starch and paprika, and roll the meat or poultry in it. This recipe works well with chicken, pork and beef. Use stewing pork or beef, and follow the recipe. You can also add more or different vegetables if you wish.

Chicken thighs, drumsticks or breast portions are all suitable. The cooking time will be quicker with breasts, or if you're going out for the day, you can leave it simmering in a crock-pot.

Ingredients for 4 servings

- 6 – 8 chicken thighs and/or drumsticks, or 4 chicken breast portions

- 2 tablespoons corn starch

- 1 tablespoon paprika

- 1 medium onion, chopped

- 1 large red pepper, deseeded and chopped

- 1 large courgette, cut into 1" chunks

- 8 mushrooms, halved

- Sea salt and freshly ground black pepper

- 1 bay leaf

- 1 small glass red wine (optional)

- 500 mls -1 liter of chicken stock

Remove the skin from the chicken portions, then make a few slashes in the meat to allow the paprika to permeate through. Now mix together the cornstarch, paprika and salt and pepper and coat the chicken in it. You may need a little more of this mixture if the portions are large. Set the chicken aside to marinade in the fridge for an hour or two.

Heat some olive oil, then soften the onions and sauté the vegetables. Place in a large casserole dish or crock-pot. Now gently fry the chicken on all sides, until it is nicely browned. Place it in the dish with the vegetables.

Add the wine to the pan, if using, and the chicken stock. Heat through, stirring around the pan to make sure any cornstarch paprika mixture remaining in the pan is incorporated into the stock. Add the bay leaf to the chicken and vegetables and pour over the stock. For chicken breasts, cook at 200 degrees C for around an hour, until the chicken is cooked through and the sauce has thickened nicely.

For thigh and drumstick portions, or stewing beef or pork, cook at 175 degrees C for 90 minutes, and then test to see if the meat is tender and cooked through. If not, return to the oven for another 30 minutes then test again. Or cook in a crock-pot on the low setting for at least 4 hours, or according to the manufacturer's instructions. Serve with wild rice or boiled new potatoes.

Chicken with lemon and olives recipe

Lemon and chicken are a classic food combination in many cuisines, and the inclusion of olives gives this dish a true Mediterranean character. Chicken thighs give the best flavor, but you can use breasts if you wish, or a combination of thighs and drumsticks.

Ingredients for 4 servings

- 8 chicken thighs, skinned and slashed

- 2 cloves of garlic

- 4 teaspoons of ground cumin

- 4 teaspoons ground paprika

- 8 tablespoons of olive oil

- 1 large onion, chopped

- 1 teaspoon of saffron

- Juice of 2 lemons

- 500 ml of chicken stock

- 2 lemons, sliced

- Medium tin of pimento stuffed olives

Place the chicken thighs into a shallow dish, after skinning and slashing them as in the previous recipe. Crush the garlic using a pestle and mortar with a pinch of salt to make it easier. Now add the cumin, paprika and freshly ground black pepper. Combine the spices with half of the olive oil and use the mixture to coat the chicken pieces. Cover and marinade in the fridge for a minimum of two to three hours.

Heat the remaining oil in a shallow flameproof casserole dish and brown the chicken, draining it on kitchen paper after cooking to remove any excess oil.

Add the onion to the pan and fry until it's soft. Add the saffron, stir and cook for a minute to release the flavor. Return the chicken to the dish and pour in the lemon juice and chicken stock. Add the lemon slices and bring everything to a simmer.

Cover the pan, reducing the heat so the mixture simmers steadily. Cook for 30 – 45 minutes, turning the chicken occasionally. Add the olives for the last 10 minutes of cooking time. If you require a thicker sauce, mix a dessertspoon of cornstarch with a little white wine and add it to the pan.

Serve the chicken with wild rice, or new potatoes and sweet corn, peas or green beans. Spinach also goes well with this dish.

Pan fried chicken marinade

Pan frying is an excellent way to cook chicken and pork quickly, sealing in the meat juices and flavors using the minimum of oil. It's also a versatile way to serve meat, because it can be accompanied by salad, baked potato, pasta, potato wedges or wild rice.

Simply mix together some olive oil, lemon juice, sea salt, black pepper and dried chili flakes. Marinate the chicken breast fillets for up to 2 hours in the fridge, then pan fry in a little olive oil or cook on the barbecue. The oily marinade will prevent the chicken from sticking to the griddle and protect it from the intense heat.

Roast chicken, Spanish style

If you fancy trying Spanish style roast chicken at home, here's a really easy recipe to try. The Spanish serve a mixture of roasted vegetables such as aubergines, carrots, courgettes, red onions, garlic cloves and potatoes with roast chicken and turkey, rather than roast or mashed potatoes and steamed vegetables and gravy. The vegetables are tossed in olive oil, seasoned with sea salt and black pepper and roasted in a large square dish for about 30 – 40 minutes on a high heat, around 225 degrees C.

Ingredients for 4 people:

- I chicken, about 1.5kg, with giblets removed

- 1 tsp paprika

- 2tbsps olive oil

- ¼ tsp turmeric

- 1 tbsp freeze dried parsley

- Sea salt and freshly ground black pepper

- 100g plum cherry tomatoes, halved

- 1 medium red pepper, cut into rough chunks

- 100g chorizo sausage, cut into 1" slices

- 600g tin of butter beans, drained

- 4 – 6 cloves of garlic, sliced

Wash the chicken thoroughly then pat it dry with kitchen paper. Cover the chicken with the olive oil and seasonings, making sure some of the mixture goes inside the cavity of the chicken to allow the flavors to penetrate right through the meat. Roast in a 180 degree C oven for an hour or so, covering the chicken loosely with foil so it doesn't dry out.

Remove the chicken from its roasting tin and pour the meat juices into a jug. Now spread the tomatoes, pepper, garlic, chorizos and butter beans on the bottom of the roasting tin. Place the chicken on top of the mixture and baste it with a little of the meat juices. Don't use too much, or the vegetables and chorizo mixture will become greasy.

Cook the chicken for another 40 minutes or so, until the juices run clear when you pierce the thigh with a skewer. Check half way through the extra cooking time in case the chicken needs basting again.

When the chicken is cooked, remove it from oven and allow it to rest while you mash together the tomatoes, butter beans, pepper and garlic.

Serve the chicken with the vegetable mash, chorizo slices and roasted vegetables. Both the chicken and the vegetable mash should be very moist, so you won't need gravy. That makes for a healthier roast, as to make a good gravy, you need some fat. While a little fat is used to baste the chicken and vegetables, it's not really a lot. If you really want potatoes with your roast chicken, boil some new potatoes in their skins.

Pork in red wine sauce recipe

Pork makes a tasty change from chicken, and if you buy loin or tenderloin, which are both widely available in the Mediterranean region, you can serve up a quick roast in a little over an hour, or cut the pork into slices and pan fry it. In Spain, sliced cured pork called lomo is available in all butchers and supermarkets, and it's ideal for this recipe. Rioja is good for cooking, as it has a mellow flavor, but any red wine that's not heavy on tannins will do. It doesn't need to be expensive.

Ingredients for 4 servings

- 8 – 12 fairly thin slices of pork, or slice up a pork loin yourself.

- Olive oil

- Salt, black pepper and a little fresh or freeze dried sage

- 2 shallots, finely chopped

- 2 small pardon or piquillo peppers, finely chopped. Or half a small green pepper if these are not available.

- I large tomato, grated

- ½ bottle of Rioja wine

Mix together the olive oil, salt and pepper and sage and coat the pork slices in the mixture. Leave in the fridge to marinate for 15 – 30 minutes.

Heat a little olive oil in a pan and brown the shallots and peppers, then reduce the heat to cook them through. This gives a unique flavor to the sauce. Now add the grated tomato and the Rioja, and bring to the boil. Simmer on a fairly high heat to reduce the sauce until it's the consistency you prefer.

While the sauce is cooking, pan fry the marinated pork, or cook it on the barbecue, using a small amount of olive oil so that it doesn't stick to the pan or dry out. Serve with the sauce and vegetables of your choice. This goes well with a mash of equal quantities of potatoes and sweet potatoes.

Marinated rabbit in white wine recipe

Rabbit is widely eaten in the Mediterranean region – on Sunday mornings you can often hear gunfire in the orange groves and woods around Europe as dutiful husbands catch Sunday lunch! Rabbit is low in fat and high in protein and flavor, and it's also inexpensive, if you can't face catching your own. This simple recipe is a great introduction to game meat, if you've always considered it too strong for your taste. If you're not too keen on garlic, use the lower amount.

Ingredients for 4 servings

- 1 rabbit, jointed and cut into portions

- 2 – 6 cloves of garlic, chopped

- 1 red onion, sliced into thin rings

- Black pepper

- 1 teaspoon each of fresh or freeze dried thyme and oregano

- 1 bay leaf

- 3 tablespoons of lemon juice or lime juice

- 250 mls dry white wine

- Salt

- A little flour for coating the rabbit before cooking

- Olive oil

Mix together all the marinade ingredients in a glass bowl and add the rabbit portions. Marinade in the fridge for 6 – 24 hours.

Drain the rabbit on kitchen paper, coat in flour and fry in the olive oil until golden brown all over. Place the rabbit in a casserole, pour over the marinade and cook at 180 degrees C until the rabbit is tender. That could be anything from 30 minutes to an hour, so check every 10 minutes and add a little more wine if the sauce is drying up. Serve with new potatoes and peas or green beans.

These recipes are typical of Mediterranean cuisine. Low in fat and calories, but high in taste, vitamin content and filling power. That's because they use fresh, high quality ingredients cooked simply from scratch. They are also very versatile, so you can change them around to suit your own personal taste or particular occasions. Now let's take a look at how the Mediterranean Diet deals with fish and seafood.

Stuffed chicken thighs braised in tomato sauce

What makes this chicken thigh recipe stand out is the rich parmesan-spinach stuffing. Not only does it add flavor to the dish but also increases the nutrient content of the dish. Should you wish to add more flavor to this recipe, you may include chicken livers in the stuffing and be engulfed in the richness of it. The usage of egg helps in binding the stuffing, so as to ensure that it does not ooze out.

This recipe for stuffed chicken thighs serves 20 people.

Ingredients:

For the stuffing:

- 2 cups of fresh breadcrumbs from whole wheat bread

- 2 cups of cooked spinach

- 1 cup of finely grated Parmesan cheese

- 4 tablespoons of finely chopped fennel fronds (optional)

- 4 tablespoons of shallots, chopped finely

- 2 large eggs, lightly beaten

- 2 tablespoons of finely minced garlic

- 1 ½ teaspoons of freshly ground black pepper, divided

- 1 teaspoon of salt, divided

- 4 teaspoons of finely chopped fresh thyme

- 20 chicken thighs, boneless, skinless and trimmed

- 8 ounces of fresh chicken livers, chopped coarsely (if required)

- 4 tablespoons of extra virgin olive oil

For the sauce:

- 1 carrot, peeled and chopped finely

- 4 cups of finely chopped onions

- 1 cup of finely diced fennel bulb

- 4 tablespoons of finely minced garlic

- 4 teaspoons of finely chopped fresh thyme

- 3 cups of dry white wine

- ½ cup of finely chopped shallots

- 2 28-ounce cans of crushed tomatoes

- 6 cups of reduced sodium chicken broth

- 4 tablespoons of finely chopped fresh basil

- ½ teaspoon of salt

- 1 teaspoon of freshly ground black pepper

First, let's get started with preparing the stuffing. Take a medium sized bowl. Add the breadcrumbs, spinach, grated parmesan, chicken livers, chopped fennel fronds, 2 tablespoons of garlic, 4 tablespoons of shallots, 1 teaspoon of pepper, ½ teaspoon of salt and thyme to the bowl and mix well. Once the ingredients have combined well, cover the bowl and place it in the refrigerator. Let the mixture rest for around 30 minutes to one hour.

Now, arrange the chicken thighs, with the skin side down, on the kitchen counter. Take around 2 to 3 tablespoons of the filling and stuff it inside a thigh. Roll the thigh slowly and use two pieces of kitchen string to secure it. Repeat the procedure with the remaining thighs. Use the remaining salt and pepper to season the thighs well.

Take a large and heavy skillet and place it over medium high heat. Add the olive oil to it and heat it. Now, lower the heat to medium and add around ¼th of the thighs to it, with the seam side down. Cook the thighs for around 7 to 10 minutes, turning twice or thrice. This should be sufficient time for the thighs to turn brown on all sides. Transfer the cooked thighs to a clean plate. Ensure that the remaining thighs are cooked in a similar fashion and transferred to the plate.

Let's get started with the sauce now. Take a large saucepan. Add the chopped onions, fennel, carrots, and 4 tablespoons of garlic and ½ cup of shallots to it and mix well. Cover the pan with lid and cook for around five minutes, stirring occasionally. This should be sufficient time for the vegetables to soften and turn brown in color. Add the white wine to the pan next and mix well. Scrape off any browned bits, with the help of a wooden spoon. Bring the mixture to a boil over medium heat. Let the mixture boil for around 6 to 8 minutes. This should be sufficient time for the liquid to get reduced by at least half. Add the chicken broth, basil, tomatoes, chicken thighs and thyme to the pan next and mix well. Crank up the heat to high and allow the mixture to boil. Once it starts boiling, lower the heat and let it simmer for around 35 to 40 minutes, stirring occasionally. This should be sufficient time for the chicken thighs to get cooked through and turn tender.

With the help of a slotted spoon, remove the thighs from the pan and cover it with foil, to keep them warm. Let the sauce simmer for some more time till it reaches the desired consistency. Season the sauce with pepper and salt and mix well.

Serve the chicken thighs warm with the sauce.

Meatballs and Spaghetti

Nothing can make your dinner special like the classic spaghetti and meatballs. This recipe uses whole wheat bread and high fiber bulgur for the meatballs. An interesting twist to this recipe is that the meatballs are baked and not fried.

This recipe for meatballs and spaghetti serves 12 people.

Ingredients:

For the meatballs:

- 2 cups of fresh breadcrumbs, made from whole wheat bread

- 1 cup of hot water

- 2/3 cups of bulgur

- 8 ounces of hot Italian sausage

- 1 teaspoon of salt

- 2 medium onions, peeled and chopped finely

- 8 ounces of lean ground beef

- 6 cloves of garlic, minced finely

- 4 large egg whites, lightly beaten

- 2 teaspoons of dried oregano

- 1 teaspoon of freshly ground black pepper

For the sauce and spaghetti:

- 8 cups of prepared marinara sauce

- 1 cup of finely chopped fresh parsley

- 2 pounds of whole wheat spaghetti

- 1 cup of finely grated parmesan cheese

Let's get started with the preparation of the meatballs first. Take a small bowl. Add the hot water and bulgur to it and mix well. Let the mixture rest for around 30 minutes. This should be sufficient time for the bulgur to absorb most of the water.

As the bulgur is resting in the water, preheat the oven to 350 degrees F. Use cooking spray to grease a rack and place it over a baking sheet, which is lined with foil.

Take a large bowl. Add the onions, egg whites, sausage, ground beef, oregano, pepper, salt, garlic, soaked bulgur and breadcrumbs to it and mix well. Shape the mixture in the form of 1-inch meatballs. You should be getting 48 meatballs out of it. Arrange the meatballs neatly on the rack and bake it for around 25 minutes. This should be sufficient time for the meatballs to get cooked well. Remove the rack from the oven at the end of 25 minutes and blot the balls well with paper towel.

Now, let's get started with the sauce and spaghetti. Place a large pot on the stove. Add some salt water to it and bring it to a boil. Add the spaghetti to it and cook it for around 8 to 10 minutes. This should be sufficient time for the spaghetti to turn tender. Drain the spaghetti and transfer it to serving plates.

Add the marinara sauce to a Dutch oven and let it simmer. Add the meatballs to it and let it cook in the sauce for around 20 minutes. Add the chopped parsley to the sauce and stir well.

Pour the sauce on top of the pasta in the serving plates. Garnish with grated Parmesan cheese and serve warm.

Herbed lamb chops with Greek couscous

This recipe uses lamb loin chops, as opposed to the traditional lamb shoulder chops, which is a healthier alternative. This is because the loin chops are not as fatty as the shoulder chops.

This recipe for herbed lamb chops with Greek couscous serves 8 people.

Ingredients:

- 2 tablespoons of finely minced garlic

- 2 cups of water

- ½ teaspoon of salt

- 2 tablespoons of fresh parsley, finely chopped

- 4 teaspoons of extra virgin olive oil

- 5 pounds of lamb loin chops, fat trimmed

- 1 cup of whole wheat couscous

- 2 medium cucumbers, peeled, deseeded and finely chopped

- 6 tablespoons of lemon juice

- 1 cup of crumbled feta

- 4 medium tomatoes, finely chopped

- 4 tablespoons of finely chopped fresh dill

Take a medium sized saucepan. Add the water to it and bring it to a boil.

As the water is boiling, take a small bowl. Add the chopped parsley, garlic and salt to it. Mix them well. Take the lamb chops. Press the parsley mixture on either sides of the lamb.

Take a large skillet. Add the olive oil to it and heat it over medium high heat. Transfer the lamb chops to the skillet and cook it for around 5 to 6 minutes. This should be sufficient time for the lamb to be cooked to medium. Place the cooked lamb aside.

As the lamb is getting cooked, add the couscous to the boiling water. Now, reduce the heat to low and let the couscous simmer in the water for around 2 minutes. At the end of two minutes, remove the pan from the heat. Cover it with a lid and allow the couscous to rest in the hot water for around 5 minutes. Fluff it with a fork at the end of 5 minutes. Transfer the fluffed couscous to a medium sized bowl. Add the chopped cucumbers, tomatoes, lemon juice, dill and feta to the bowl. Ensure that the ingredients are mixed well.

Serve the lamb warm with the couscous salad.

Chapter 5:
Fish and Seafood

Fish and seafood is at the very core of the Mediterranean Diet. Often, it's either steamed, baked, poached or cooked on the barbecue, rather than being coated in batter or breadcrumbs, so it's high in flavor and Omega-3 fatty acids, and low in calories and fat. Omega-3 is good for your heart and they help keep your joints working well, so they are very important to good health. Try and eat at least 2 – 3 servings of oily fish such as salmon, tuna, sardines and mackerel each week. Cod and haddock are also excellent, healthy choices. Here are a few ideas for cooking fish the Mediterranean way.

Baked fish with tomatoes recipe

For a light, tasty summer fish dish with a difference, try this recipe. It's quick and easy to cook, but the flavor is divine and so very Mediterranean! It's also low in fat, so it's healthy as well as delicious.

The beauty of this recipe is you can make it with almost any white fish; cod, hake halibut and plaice all work well. As the cooking time is so short, go for a tailpiece if using hake or cod. Serve with a baked potato or potato wedges and peas or green beans. If you prefer it, you can serve with a large salad and a basket of fresh crusty bread.

Ingredients for 2 people

- 2 fish fillets, 250 – 350 grams in total weight

- 1 large ripe tomato, sliced. (A beef tomato is ideal for this)

- Olive oil

- Balsamic vinegar

- Sea salt and freshly ground black pepper

- Fresh or freeze dried parsley

Heat the oven to 200 degrees C. Layer the tomato in a shallow ovenproof dish, drizzle with olive oil and balsamic vinegar and season generously.

Place the fish on top of the tomatoes and sprinkle with the parsley. Bake for around 15 minutes. Test with a fork to see if it's cooked. The fish should be nice and white and should flake easily. If necessary, allow a little extra cooking time, but not so long that the fish becomes tough and rubbery.

Use a fish slice and a spatula or and carefully lift each piece of fish together with its bed of tomatoes. Pour the remaining cooking juices over the fish. Serve with a wedge of lemon or lime.

Oven cooked sea bass recipe

Sea bass is a lovely meaty fish with a delicate flavor that is best baked to bring out the best of it. This recipe uses a bed of vegetables to accompany the fish, and the combination of fish and Mediterranean vegetables works really well.

- 2 sea bass cleaned and descaled – the fishmonger will do this for you if you ask.

- 2 medium-sized potatoes sliced fairly thickly and parboiled for 5 minutes. For extra color, texture and fiber, leave the skin on the potatoes.

- 1 red pepper, cut into chunks

- 1 courgette, sliced fairly thickly

- 1 aubergine, cut into chunks

- 1 red onion, cut into wedges

- 1 large or 2 smaller vine tomatoes, cut into wedges. (or 1 beef tomato)

- 1 – 2 chopped garlic cloves

- Extra virgin olive oil

- Seasoning

Preheat the oven to 200 C, then drizzle olive oil over the base of a shallow ovenproof dish. Spread the potatoes over the bottom of the dish, then top with garlic, seasoning and other vegetables – except the tomatoes. Cook in oven for 15 minutes.

Slash skin on both sides of the fish, season with salt, pepper and freshly squeezed lemon or lime juice. Place fish on top of vegetables and surround with tomatoes. This helps to keep the fish and the rest of the vegetables moist. Cook for about 30 minutes, until the fish is cooked – but not overcooked – and the vegetables are just starting to crisp and go brown at the edges. Sprinkle with fresh or freeze dried parsley to serve.

Pan fried fresh tuna marinade

While canned tuna is just as good as fresh tuna from a nutrition point of view, the flavor is very different. Fresh tuna is meatier in texture and has a much stronger taste. It's best served simply, pan fried after marinating in a mixture of equal parts of olive oil and lime juice, seasoned with black pepper and fresh parsley. Coat the tuna with the marinade and store in the fridge for 20 – 45 minutes before pan frying in a little olive oil. Serve with a big salad, potato wedges or homemade coleslaw. Try making the coleslaw with red cabbage for a change.

Cod with lemon and parsley recipe

Here's a simple but tasty recipe for cod, using fresh lemons, which are the perfect natural partner for fish. You could also use any other firm-fleshed white fish, such as haddock or hake

Ingredients to serve 2 People

- 2 cod fillets

- Seasoned flour

- 1 large lemon, or 2 small ones

- 1 tbsp olive oil

- 1 tbsp of fresh or freeze dried parsley

- Salt and freshly milled pepper

Coat the fish fillets with seasoned flour, then squeeze the juice from the lemon. Make sure it is at room temperature, as this will yield more juice

Heat the oil and cook the fish for about 5 minutes on each side. Now add the lemon juice and seasoning to the pan. Allow the sauce to bubble and thicken for a minute or two, then stir in the parsley. That's all you need to do!

Serve with new potatoes and peas, green beans or salad.

Mussels in spicy sauce recipe

This is a tasty recipe with a spicy sauce, which makes a change from the traditional mussels in garlic and white wine.

Some people are concerned about getting food poisoning from mussels, but there are three foolproof ways to ensure you don't eat 'bad' mussels. If any of the mussels are open, tap the shell with the handle of a knife. If the shell closes, the mussel is safe to eat. Discard any that don't close, or any that bob around on the surface of the water when you wash them. Finally, any mussels which don't open after 5 minutes of cooking should also be discarded.

Ingredients for 2 people as a light lunch or 4 as starters

- 1 kg mussels

- 1 glass white wine

- 1 chili pepper, chopped

- 4 cloves of garlic, crushed or finely chopped

- 2 shallots, finely chopped

- 500g large ripe tomatoes, grated

- Freshly milled black pepper

- 1 tablespoon of fresh or freeze dried parsley

- Extra virgin olive oil

- Wash mussels well and pull out the 'beards.'

Heat the wine in a large lidded pan, then cook the mussels until most of them are open - 5 minutes or less.

Remove the mussels with a slotted spoon and set aside. Strain the cooking liquid to remove any sand or grit. Return the liquid to pan and boil until it's reduced by half.

Heat some olive oil in a pan and add the shallots, garlic and chili peppers. Cook for about 5 minutes until soft. Now add the mussel liquid and grated tomatoes and heat thoroughly. Allow the sauce to stand for a few minutes to allow flavors to blend. Taste and season with pepper if necessary.

Remove the empty half of the shell from each mussel, and then stir them into the sauce until they are well coated. Sprinkle with parsley and serve with fresh crusty bread.

These tasty recipes will help you to get your servings of fish every week, as well as showing you how to incorporate more fish into your diet by using simple, healthy recipes.

Stuffed sardines

These are not just fried sardines but sardines stuffed with cheese. This would make do for an interesting first course.

This recipe for stuffed sardines serves 12 people.

Ingredients:

- 24 medium fresh sardines

- ½ cup of shredded Pecorino Romano cheese

- ½ cup of part-skim ricotta cheese

- ½ cup of finely chopped fresh parsley

- 6 large eggs, divided

- ½ cup of fresh breadcrumbs

- Zest of 2 lemons, plus lemon wedges for serving

- 1 teaspoon of freshly ground black pepper, divided

- 1 teaspoon of salt, divided

- 2/3 cup of all-purpose flour

- 3 cups of extra virgin olive oil

- 4 cups of panko breadcrumbs

Ensure that the sardines are gutted. Leave the head and tail on, while you prepare the sardines.

Take a medium sized bowl. Add the shredded Pecorino Romano cheese, ricotta cheese, breadcrumbs, 2 eggs, fresh breadcrumbs, parsley, ½ teaspoon of pepper, lemon zest and ½ teaspoon of salt to it and mix well. Ensure that all the ingredients are mixed well.

Take the sardines and rinse them well. Use paper towels to pat them dry. Use the remaining salt and pepper to season the insides of the sardines. Take two teaspoons of the cheese mixture and stuff it carefully inside each sardine.

Take a shallow dish. Add the flour to it. Take another shallow dish. Lightly beat the remaining eggs and add it to the second dish. Place the panko breadcrumbs in a third shallow dish. Take a stuffed sardine and dip it in the flour first. Dip it in the eggs next and finally in the panko breadcrumbs. Ensure that the remaining sardines are coated in this fashion.

Fish couscous with onion T'faya

This is a Moroccan specialty, which is well known for its vibrant flavors. The raisins add a touch of sweetness to this halibut dish.

This recipe of fish couscous serves 16 people.

Ingredients:

- 8 tablespoons of extra virgin olive oil, divided

- 1 cup of raisins

- 1 cup of slivered or thinly sliced almonds

- 4 tablespoons of butter

- 4 teaspoons of salt

- 16 saffron threads

- 2 teaspoons of ground turmeric

- 1 teaspoon of ground allspice

- 1 teaspoon of ground nutmeg

- 5 pounds Pacific halibut, skins removed and cut into 2 inch wide chunks

- 2 teaspoons of ground ginger

- 1 teaspoon of ground cinnamon

- 6 large onions, peeled and sliced thinly

- 2 tablespoons of sugar

- 4 2/3 cups of reduced sodium chicken broth, divided

- 1 teaspoon of freshly ground black pepper, plus more to taste

- 2 tablespoons of canola oil

- 2 cups of whole wheat couscous

- Water

Take a small bowl first. Add the raisins to it and pour some warm water over it. Let the raisins soak in the water for around ten minutes. Drain them at the end of ten minutes and keep aside.

Take a mortar. Add the saffron and salt to it and crush it well using the pestle. Keep crushing till you get a coarse powder. Transfer the powder to another small bowl. Add the turmeric, ginger, nutmeg, allspice, pepper and cinnamon to the bowl and mix well.

Now, add four tablespoons of olive oil and butter to a Dutch oven and heat it over medium heat. Add the spice mixture to it and cook it, while stirring continuously. Keep cooking till the consistency of the spice mixture is foamy. Now, add the sugar, onions and soaked raisins to the spice mixture and mix well. Cook the mixture for around 20 to 25 minutes. This should be sufficient time for the onions to turn light brown in color. Pour around 2 cups of the chicken broth into the oven. Add the fish pieces to the mixture next. Cover with lid and cook the fish for around 8 to 10 minutes in the onion mixture. This should be sufficient time for the fish to turn flaky. Once the fish starts flaking, remove the dish from the heat. Season well with pepper and cover it. Keep it aside.

As the fish is getting cooked, take a small skillet. Add the canola oil to it and heat it over medium high heat. Add the slivered almonds to it and cook it for around 1 minute. This should be sufficient time for the almonds to turn golden. Remove them from the skillet and place them on paper towels, to drain off any excess oil.

Take a small saucepan. Add the remaining olive oil and chicken broth to it and mix well. Bring the mixture to a boil. As it starts boiling, add the couscous to it and stir once. Cover the saucepan with a lid and remove it from the heat. Allow the couscous to rest in the saucepan for around five minutes, before fluffing it with a fork.

Transfer the cooked couscous to serving plates. Arrange the fish pieces and the onion mixture on top of the couscous. Garnish the dish with the almonds and serve immediately.

Greek Fava with grilled squid

Fava is nothing but a bean puree made from yellow split peas. Paired with grilled squid, this is a refreshing and simple seafood dish. The raw onions, olive oil and lemon juice not only add an element of zing to this dish but also succeed in highlighting squid as the hero of the dish.

This recipe of fava with grilled squid serves 12 people.

Ingredients:

- 2 small red onions, peeled and chopped finely

- 1 ½ cups of yellow split peas

- 4 cups of vegetable broth, plus more as needed

- 6 tablespoons of extra virgin olive oil, divided

- 1 ½ teaspoons of salt, divided

- 4 tablespoons of lemon juice

- 24 ounces of squid, cleaned well

- 4 tablespoons of finely chopped fresh parsley

- ½ teaspoons of freshly ground black pepper, plus more to taste

- 2 lemons, cut into wedges

Take the split peas first and rinse them well under running water. This will ensure that the peas are free from grit and pebbles.

Take a large saucepan and place it over medium heat. Add 2 tablespoons of olive oil to the pan and heat it. Add the chopped onions to the pan and cook it for around 5 minutes. This should be sufficient time for the onions to soften. Add the split peas to the pan next and toss well so as to coat. Pour the vegetable broth into the pan next and bring the mixture to a boil, over high heat. Once the mixture starts boiling, reduce the heat and cover the pan with a lid. Let the mixture simmer for around 45 minutes to 1 hour, stirring occasionally. This should be sufficient time for the peas to turn tender and for the liquid to get absorbed. If the peas begin to disintegrate easily, it is an indication that they are cooked and tender. In case, the liquid gets absorbed before the peas could get cooked, add some more broth to the pan.

As the broth is getting cooked in the pan, take the squid. Cut the squid into rings that are half an inch thick. Do not chop the tentacles. Take a medium sized bowl. Add the squid rings and tentacles to it. Add 1 teaspoon of salt, 3 teaspoons of oil and ½ teaspoon of pepper to the bowl and mix well. Keep it aside.

Transfer the cooked peas to the bowl of a food processor. Add around 3 teaspoons of oil, ½ teaspoon of salt and lemon juice to it. Pulse the ingredients till the consistency of the mixture is that of a mash. Spread the peas puree neatly on the serving plates.

Preheat the grill to medium high.

Thread the squid tentacles and rings on skewers. Gently, oil the grill rack. Place the squid on the rack and grill it for around 4 minutes, turning once. This should be sufficient time for the squid to turn firm and remain tender. Once the squid has cooked through, remove the skewers from the grill. Remove the squid from the skewers and arrange neatly on top of the fava. Drizzle with oil. Season the squid well with pepper and salt. Sprinkle the parsley on top of the squid. Serve warm with lemon wedges.

Chapter 6:
Sides, Appetizers and Salad Recipes

Let us have a look at some interesting and healthy recipes for appetizers, salads and sides in this chapter.

Butternut squash pilaf

What makes this brown rice dish interesting is the addition of grated butternut squash. Not only does it add color to the dish but also packs the dish with nutrients. This Greek recipe was originally made with pumpkins, but was later modified to replace it with butternut squash, considering the availability of this vegetable in the U.S. If you cannot get your hands on pilaf rice, which is nothing but polished and short grain rice, you can use brown rice.

This recipe for butternut squash pilaf serves 4 people.

Ingredients:

- 1 pound butternut squash

- ½ large red onion, chopped finely

- 1 tablespoon of water

- 1 ½ tablespoons of extra virgin olive oil

- ½ clove of garlic, minced finely

- ½ cup of instant boiled brown rice

- ½ tablespoon of tomato paste

- ½ 14 ounce can of vegetable broth

- 1 tablespoon of fresh oregano, finely chopped

- ¼ cup of white wine

- ¼ cup of fennel fronds, chopped finely

- ½ teaspoon of salt

- Freshly ground black pepper, to taste

- Pinch of ground cinnamon

First, take the butternut squash. Peel the squash and cut in halves. Remove the seeds from the center of the halves. With the help of a box grater, grate the halves. Keep aside.

Take a large non-stick skillet. Place it over a medium low heat. Add the olive oil to it and heat it. Now, add the chopped onion and garlic to the skillet and stir well for around 10 to 12 minutes. This should be sufficient time for the onions and garlic to soften and turn translucent. As the onions and garlic are getting cooked in the skillet, take a small bowl. Add the water and tomato paste to it and mix well. Stir in the tomato paste into the skillet next and stir well.

Next, add the instant rice to the skillet and stir well. Ensure that the rice is coated well with the mixture. Add in the grated squash to the skillet next and stir well. Ensure that the mixture is reduced well.

Once the mixture has reduced well, increase the heat to medium high. Pour in the vegetable broth and white wine next and stir well. Cover the skillet with a lid and bring the mixture to a boil. Once the mixture begins to boil, reduce the heat to medium low and cook for another 25 to 30 minutes, stirring once or twice. This should be sufficient time for the rice to absorb most of the liquid and the squash to turn tender.

Now, add the chopped fennel fronds, salt, cinnamon, oregano and pepper to the skillet and stir well. Remove the skillet from the heat and allow the mixture to rest, covered, for another five minutes. Serve hot.

Lima bean spread with herbs and cumin

This recipe is an opportunity for you to use the lima beans in an interesting fashion. This refreshing dish is packed with vibrant flavors, thanks to the inclusion of spices and fresh herbs.

This recipe of lima bean spread serves 3 people.

Ingredients:

- 8 cloves of garlic, crushed and peeled

- 2 10-ounce packages of frozen lima beans

- 2 tablespoons of finely chopped fresh cilantro

- 4 tablespoons of extra virgin olive oil

- ½ teaspoon of finely crushed red pepper

- 2 teaspoons of ground cumin

- 2 teaspoons of salt, to taste

- 8 teaspoons of lemon juice

- 2 tablespoons of finely chopped fresh mint

- Freshly ground black pepper, to taste

- 2 tablespoons of finely chopped fresh dill

- Water

Take a large saucepan and fill it water. Add one teaspoon of salt to the water and bring it to a boil. As the water starts boiling, add the lima beans, crushed red pepper and garlic to the pan and stir well. Cook the mixture for ten minutes. This should be sufficient time for the beans to turn tender. Once the beans have turned tender, remove the saucepan from the heat and allow the mixture to cool.

Now, drain the beans and garlic. Transfer the cooked beans and garlic to the bowl of a food processor. Add the olive oil, cumin, lemon juice, pepper and salt to the processor. Pulse until the mixture is smooth. Transfer the mixture to a bowl.

Add the chopped dill, mint and cilantro to the bowl next and stir well. Serve immediately.

Roasted root vegetables with chermoula

This recipe is an interesting take on winter squash and root vegetables. The inclusion of Moroccan spices adds an interesting flavor profile to this dish. This recipe serves 12 people.

Ingredients:

- 6 cloves of garlic, finely minced

- 2 medium baking potatoes

- ½ cup of extra virgin olive oil

- 4 medium carrots

- 4 teaspoons of ground cumin

- 2 medium turnips

- 4 teaspoons of sweet Hungarian paprika

- 2 teaspoons of salt

- 2 medium rutabagas

- 16 ounces of butternut squash

- 2 medium sweet potatoes

First, let us get started with preparing the vegetables, which are the core ingredients of this dish. Take the turnips first. Peel their skins off and cut them into one-inch chunks. Take the sweet potatoes next. Peel their skins off and cut them into one-inch chunks. Now, take the baking potatoes. Peel their skins off and cut them into one-inch chunks. Take the rutabagas next. Remove their skins and chop them into smaller pieces. Take the carrots next. Wash them well and chop them into small pieces. Finally, take the butternut squash. Peel the squash and cut in halves. Remove the seeds from the center of the halves.

Now that the vegetables are prepared, preheat the oven to 425 degrees F.

Add the cumin, olive oil, salt, garlic and paprika to a food processor and blend till the mixture turns smooth.

Take a large roasting pan now. Add the vegetables to the pan. Pour the spice oil mixture on top of the vegetables and mix well. Place the pan in the oven and cook the vegetables for around 45 to 50 minutes. This should be sufficient time for the vegetables to get roasted well. Serve immediately.

Roasted eggplant and feta dip

The addition of fresh jalapeno and cayenne pepper gives a kick to this classic Greek dish. If you are doing this dish when eggplants are not in season, there is a high probability that these eggplants were watered heavily. This means that there will be lots of seeds, which can make the dish, taste a tad bitter to your liking. This can be easily remedied by including a little sugar to the dish. Toast some pita crisps and serve it with this!

This recipe of roasted eggplant and feta dip serves 12 people.

Ingredients:

- ¼ cup of extra virgin olive oil

- 1 medium eggplant

- ½ cup of crumbled feta cheese

- ½ cup of chopped red onion

- 2 tablespoons of lemon juice

- 1 small jalapeno, deseeded and minced finely

- ¼ teaspoon of cayenne pepper, to taste

- 1 small red bell pepper, chopped finely

- 1 tablespoon of chopped parsley

- 2 tablespoons of finely chopped fresh basil

- ¼ teaspoon of salt

- Pinch of sugar, if required

First position oven rack around 6 inches from the heat. Preheat the broiler.

Use foil to line a baking pan. Now, arrange the eggplant on the pan. To vent steam, poke some holes on the eggplant. Place the pan in the broiler and cook the eggplant for around 14 to 18 minutes. Ensure that you turn the eggplant every five minutes. This should be sufficient time for the skin to get charred and the flesh to get cooked. To check if the eggplant has cooked through, insert a knife into the flesh. If your knife goes in smoothly, it means your eggplant is cooked through. Transfer the cooked eggplant to a cutting board for it to cool.

As the eggplant is cooling, take a medium bowl. Add the lemon juice to the bowl. Now, cut the eggplant in half, lengthwise and scoop out the flesh. Add the flesh to the bowl and mix it with the lemon juice. This will prevent the discoloring of the eggplant. Add the olive oil to the bowl and stir well.

Add the crumbled feta, chopped onions, bell pepper, jalapeno, parsley, basil, salt and cayenne pepper to the bowl and mix well. Taste and add sugar, if the mixture is too bitter. Transfer it to serving bowls and serve with toasted pita crisps.

Orange, olive and anchovy salad

This Italian salad is not only refreshing but also easy to make. This makes an exciting first course and tastes better, when served with roasted chicken.

This salad recipe serves 8 people.

Ingredients:

- 2 small red onions, sliced thinly

- 12 anchovy fillets

- 8 small oranges

- 2 tablespoons of fresh lemon juice

- 32 oil-cured Kalamata olives, pits removed and cut in halves

- ¼ teaspoon of freshly ground black pepper, to taste

- 4 teaspoons of finely minced fennel fronds, for garnish

- 6 tablespoons of extra virgin olive oil

Take the oranges first. Peel their skins off and remove the piths. Slice the oranges into thin slices. This will help you to get all the juice.

Now, arrange the slices neatly on a serving platter. Reserve the orange juice for later. Arrange the onion slices on top of the orange slices. Now, arrange the cured olives on top of the onion slices. Finally, arrange the anchovy fillets on top of the olives.

Pour the lemon juice and orange juice on top of the salad.

Drizzle salad with the olive oil. Sprinkle the freshly ground black pepper on top of the salad.

Allow the salad to rest, at room temperature, for around 30 minutes. This should be sufficient time for the flavors to get infused well. Once the salad has rested well, garnish it with the minced fennel fronds. Serve immediately.

Warm arugula bread salad

When prepared with mature arugula, this salad is absolutely refreshing. However, if you can't get your hands on mature arugula, baby arugula also works fine. Serve this warm salad with turkey sausage or grilled steak!

This recipe serves 8 people.

Ingredients:

- 2 cups of cherry tomatoes, cut in halves

- 6 tablespoons of extra virgin olive oil, divided

- 16 cups of arugula

- 4 slices of crusty whole wheat bread, chopped into even sized cubes

- 2 tablespoons of finely minced garlic

- ¼ teaspoon of freshly ground black pepper

- 4 tablespoons of balsamic vinegar

- ¼ teaspoon of salt

- ½ cup of grated Parmesan cheese

Take a large non-stick skillet. Add four tablespoons of olive oil to it and heat it over medium high heat. Add the bread cubes to it and cook it for around 5 to 6 minutes, stirring occasionally. This should be sufficient time for the bread cubes to turn crisp and brown in color.

Now, add the halved cherry tomatoes and arugula to the skillet and cook for another minute. This should be sufficient time for the arugula leaves to wilt. Once the leaves have wilted, push the mixture to one side of the skillet. Add the remaining olive oil to the empty side of the skillet. Add the minced garlic to the skillet and cook it for around fifteen seconds. Now, mix the garlic with the bread mixture. Remove the skillet from the heat.

Season the salad well with pepper and salt. Drizzle the salad with balsamic vinegar and toss to ensure that the ingredients are combined well. Garnish the salad with grated Parmesan cheese and serve warm.

Chapter 7:
Dessert Recipes

In this chapter, let us look at some exciting dessert recipes.

Apricot bulgur pudding cake and custard sauce

What makes this recipe stand out is the interesting combination of bulgur and cake.

This recipe for apricot bulgur pudding cake serves 8 people.

Ingredients:

For the cake:

- 1/3 cup of granulated sugar

- ½ cup of toasted pistachios, finely chopped

- ½ cup of finely chopped dried apricots

- 1 cup of orange juice, freshly squeezed

- 1 cup of water

- 1 teaspoon of orange zest, finely slivered

- ½ cup of bulgur

- 2/3 cup of low fat milk

- 2 large eggs, separated

- 2 tablespoons of brown sugar

For the sauce:

- 1 tablespoon of sugar

- ½ cup of low fat milk

- 1 teaspoon of kirsch

- 1 large egg yolk, beaten lightly

Let's first get started with the custard sauce. Take a small bowl and place a fine mesh sieve over it. Add some water to a double broiler and let it simmer in the bottom layer of the broiler. Now, add the sugar, egg yolk and milk to the upper of the broiler and whisk well. Stir the mixture well over the hot water. Adjust the heat, as and when required, to ensure that a gentle simmer is maintained and cook the sauce for around 4 to 8 minutes. This should be sufficient time for the temperature to touch 160 degrees F and the sauce to thicken. Pour the sauce through the sieve. Add the kirsch to the bowl and whisk well. Cover the bowl with plastic wrap and place it in the refrigerator. Let it rest there for around 1-½ hours. This should be sufficient time for the sauce to chill.

Take a medium saucepan and place it on the stove. Add the orange zest, apricots, sugar, water and orange juice to it and mix well. Allow the mixture to boil. Once it starts boiling, reduce the heat and let it simmer for around 10 minutes, stirring occasionally. This should be sufficient time for the apricots to get cooked and turn tender. Now, add in the bulgur and crank up the heat to high. Once again, bring the mixture to a boil. Once it starts boiling, reduce the heat to low and let the mixture simmer for around 20 minutes, stirring occasionally. This should be sufficient time for the bulgur to turn tender. Remove the saucepan from the heat and let it cool, uncovered, for around 10 minutes.

Now, position a rack in the center of the oven. Preheat the oven to 350 degrees F.

Take a large bowl. Add the milk and egg yolks to it and whisk well. Now, add in the bulgur mixture and whisk well.

Take a medium sized bowl. Add the egg whites to it and beat it, with the help of a mixer on medium high speed. Keep beating until stiff peaks form. Now, add the bulgur mixture to the bowl and mix well.

Now, take an 8 inch square baking dish. Transfer the batter to it. Using a sieve, sprinkle the brown sugar evenly over the batter. Place the baking dish in the roasting pan and transfer it to the oven. Fill half the roasting pan with hot water, till it comes around halfway up to the sides of the baking dish. Bake the cake for around 30 to 40 minutes. This should be sufficient time for the cake to puff and turn golden in color.

At the end of 40 minutes, remove the baking dish from the hot water. Place it on a wire rack to allow the cake to cool. Cut the cake into 8 equal servings and transfer it to serving plates. Divide the custard sauce among the 8 servings. Garnish the pieces with the chopped pistachios and serve immediately.

Orange hazelnut cake

This is a very light and fluffy cake, completely wheat free. This recipe is a Jewish specialty in the Asian side of Istanbul.

This recipe for orange hazelnut cake serves 8 to 10 people.

Ingredients:

For the cake:

- 5 large eggs, separated

- 2 ¼ cups of hazelnut flour

- 1 cup of superfine sugar

For the syrup:

- 2 ½ tablespoons of orange juice

- Finely grated zest from 1 orange

- 2 ½ tablespoons of orange flower water

- 1 ¼ cups of superfine sugar

- 2/3 cup of water

To serve:

- 2 tablespoons of confectioner's sugar

- Pulp from 4 passion fruits

- 1 1/3 cups of Greek style yogurt

Preheat the oven to 350 degrees F.

First, let us get started with preparing the syrup. Take a saucepan and add the water to it. Bring it to a boil. Add the sugar and orange juice to the pan and allow it to simmer for around 10 to 12 minutes. This should be sufficient time for the sugar to dissolve and the mixture to turn syrupy. Remove the saucepan from the heat. Allow the syrup to cool. Once the syrup has cooled enough, add the orange zest and orange flower water to the bowl and mix well.

Now, let us get on with preparing the cake. Add the egg yolks and sugar to the bowl of an electric mixer and blend it on high speed. Blend it till the mixture turns thick and pale. Now, fold in the hazelnut flour. Take a small bowl. Add the egg whites to it and whisk it well. Keep whisking till the egg whites turn glossy and stiff. Add them to the hazelnut mixture and mix well.

Use cooking spray to grease a loaf pan and use parchment paper to line it. Transfer the batter to the pan. Place the pan in the oven and let it bake for around 30 minutes. This should be sufficient time for the cake to turn lightly golden in color. At the end of thirty minutes, remove the cake from the oven. Pour the orange syrup on top of the cake and spread it evenly.

Take another small bowl. Add the confectioner's sugar, passion fruit pulp and yogurt to it and mix well. Serve it with the cake.

Cornmeal Rosemary cake with orange glaze and pine nuts

This recipe is an exciting projection of the flavors of rosemary and cornmeal, two completely different ingredients.

This recipe for cornmeal rosemary cake serves 8 to 10 people.

Ingredients:

For the cake:

- 1 ½ cups of all-purpose flour

- Soft butter

- 1 1/3 cups of granulated sugar

- ¾ cup of finely ground yellow cornmeal

- 1 tablespoon of fresh rosemary, finely chopped

- 1/3 cup of toasted pine nuts, coarsely chopped

- 1 teaspoon of baking powder

- ¼ teaspoon of kosher salt

- 1 tablespoon of finely grated orange zest

- 4 large eggs

- 2/3 cup of mascarpone

- ½ cup of unsalted butter, melted

For the orange syrup:

- 3 tablespoons of granulated sugar

- ½ cup of fresh orange juice

For the orange glaze:

- 1 ½ cups of sifted confectioners' sugar

- 2 tablespoons of fresh orange juice

- 5 tablespoons of heavy cream

- 1 tablespoon of whole fresh rosemary leaves, stems removed

- 1 teaspoon of grated orange zest

Let us first begin with the cake. Place a rack in the center of the oven. Heat the oven to 350 degrees F. Use butter to grease a 9x2 inch round cake pan. Line the pan with the parchment paper and butter the paper as well.

Take a medium sized bowl. Add the cornmeal, pine nuts, flour, orange zest, rosemary, salt and baking powder to it and whisk well.

Take a large bowl. Add the mascarpone to it and whisk it well. This should loosen it. Add the eggs to the bowl, one at a time. Whisk continuously for the eggs to combine with the mascarpone. Now, add the sugar to the bowl and whisk well till the consistency of the mixture is smooth. With the help of a rubber spatula, add the flour mixture to the bowl and fold in well. Keep mixing till all the ingredients combine well and the consistency of the batter is smooth. Now, add the melted butter to the batter and mix well.

Now, transfer the batter to the cake pan. Ensure that the batter is spread in an even fashion. Place it in the oven and bake it for around 40 to 45 minutes. This should be sufficient time for the top layer of the cake to turn golden brown in color. To check if the cake has cooked well, insert a skewer in the center of the cake. If it comes out clean, it means your cake is good to go. Make sure that the sides of the cake are not sticking to the pan.

As the cake is getting baked, let us get on with making the orange syrup. Take a small saucepan and place it over medium heat. Add the sugar and orange juice to it and cook it for few minutes, while stirring occasionally. Keep cooking till the sugar dissolves completely in the orange juice. Once the sugar dissolves, remove the pan from the heat.

Once the cake has cooked, place the pan in the wire rack and let it cool for around 5 minutes. Take a small knife and run it around the cake. Take an inverted plate and place it over the cake pan. With a kitchen towel to protect your hands, carefully invert the cake onto the plate. Once the cake has slid over to the plate, peel off the parchment paper. Now, place another inverted plate on top of the cake and invert the cake again. Remove the plate placed on top of the cake. Now, take a toothpick and poke several holes on top of the cake. As the cake is warm, brush it gently with the orange syrup. Keep brushing for few minutes to let the syrup sink in. Once all the syrup has been used up, allow the cake to cool.

As the cake is cooling, let us get on with the preparation of the orange glaze. Take a small saucepan and add some water to it. Bring it to a boil. Keep a bowl of ice water handy as well. Place the rosemary leaves in a small sieve. Place the sieve in the boiling water and blanch the leaves for around one minute. At the end of 1 minute, drain the rosemary leaves and place the sieve in the ice water. Now, drain the leaves again and arrange them neatly on a paper towel. Allow the leaves to dry. As the leaves are drying, take another bowl. Add the cream, confectioner's sugar and orange juice to it and whisk well. Keep whisking till the consistency of the mixture is smooth. Now, add the blanched rosemary leaves and zest to the bowl and mix well.

Once the cake has cooled, transfer it to a rack placed over a baking sheet. Pour the orange glaze carefully on top of the cake and allow it to drip off the sides. To ensure that the glaze completely coats the cake, tilt the wire rack gently. Transfer the cake to a cake plate, when the glaze is still wet. Allow the cake to cool for at least an hour. Once the cake has cooled enough, cut into wedges and serve.

Pear strudel

This is a crispy take on the classic pear strudel. The combination of nuts and pears makes it different from your conventional pear strudel.

This recipe for pear strudel serves 6 to 8 people.

Ingredients:

- 2 cups of granulated sugar

- 2 cups of water

- ½ vanilla bean, deseeded and cut in half lengthwise

- 1 teaspoon of pure vanilla extract

- 4 slices of fresh ginger

- 2 strips of lemon zest

- 2 tablespoons of lemon juice

- 1/3 cup of golden raisins

- 2 tablespoons of Cognac

- 4 ripe Bartlett pears

- 1/3 cup of whole almonds, with their skins on

- 4 sheets of frozen phyllo dough, thawed

- ½ cup of unsalted butter, melted

- ½ cup of coarsely crushed amaretti cookies

- Confectioners' sugar, for sprinkling purposes

Take the pears first. Peel their skins off first. Cut them in halves and remove the core and seeds. Cut each pear lengthwise into 8 slices each.

Take a medium saucepan and place it over high heat. Add the water and sugar to it and mix well. Allow the mixture to boil. Stir continuously to ensure that the sugar dissolves in the water. Once the sugar has dissolved, add the lemon zest, ginger and vanilla bean to the pan and mix well. Lower the heat and allow the mixture to simmer for around 10 minutes. Now, add the lemon juice, vanilla extract and pear slices to the pan. Cover the pan with a lid and poach the pears for around 15 minutes. This should be sufficient time for the pears to turn soft. At the end of 15 minutes, remove the pan from the heat and transfer its contents to a bowl. Place the bowl in the refrigerator and let the pears cool for at least 2 hours. As the pears are resting, take a small bowl. Add the raisins to it and pour the cognac on top of it. Place the bowl in the refrigerator and let the raisins soak for at least 2 hours.

Heat the oven to 325 degrees F. Arrange the almonds on a small baking sheet and toast them for around 12 minutes. This should be sufficient time for the almonds to turn golden brown in the center. Allow the almonds to cool. Once they have cooled enough, chop them coarsely and keep aside.

Now, increase the heat to 400 degrees F. Place the pear slices in a colander. This should drain off any syrup.

Place a clean and damp dish towel on the kitchen counter. Lay the phyllo sheets on top of the dishtowel. Cover the sheets with another damp dishtowel. This will ensure that the pastry sheets do not dry out. Now, take a parchment that is larger than the phyllo sheets and arrange it on the kitchen counter. Take out two phyllo sheets and arrange them on top of the parchment, with the longest end facing towards you. Brush the sheets generously with the melted butter. Sprinkle the chopped almonds on top of the sheets. Now, take out another two sheets and arrange them on top of the parchment. Brush these sheets with the melted butter and sprinkle almonds on top of them.

Now, take the Amaretti crumbs and sprinkle them about 2 inches wide, near the edge closest to you. Arrange the pear slices on top of the crumbs. Sprinkle the raisins on top of the pears.

Start at the edge closest to you and roll up the strudel, with the help of the parchment. Place the strudel on a baking sheet, which is lined with parchment paper. Use a serrated knife to score the top of the strudel. Ensure that the cuts are 2 inches apart. Place the baking sheet in the oven and bake the strudel for around 20 minutes. At the end of 20 minutes, reduce the temperature to 350 degrees F. Continue to bake the strudel for another 10 to 15 minutes. This should be sufficient time for the pastry to turn deep golden brown in color. Allow the strudel to cool for a few minutes. Sprinkle the confectioners' sugar on top of the strudel before serving.

Pumpkin Pie Flan

This is a take on the classic Spanish custard, which is covered with caramel sauce. What makes this dessert stand out from the classic is the inclusion of the spices in the sauce!

This recipe for pumpkin pie flan serves 8 people.

Ingredients:

- 2/3 cups of granulated sugar

- ½ cup of whole milk

- ¼ cup of evaporated milk

- 2 large eggs

- 2 large egg yolks

- 1 teaspoon of vanilla extract

- 1 teaspoon of ground cinnamon

- ½ teaspoon of ground nutmeg

- ¾ cup of canned pumpkin

- 4 cups of water

Heat the oven to 350 degrees F. Take 8 ramekins and arrange them neatly on a 9x13 inch-baking pan. Use cooking spray to coat these ramekins.

Take a small saucepan. Add 1/3 cup of the granulated sugar to it and heat it over medium heat. Keep stirring continuously till the sugar melts. Heat it for around 7 minutes till the sugar turns into a medium brown caramel. Now, quickly transfer around 2 teaspoons of the caramel to each of the ramekins. Keep swirling as you spoon the caramel to ensure that it does not harden. Keep the ramekins aside.

Take a medium sized saucepan and place it over medium heat. Add the evaporated milk and whole milk to it and mix well. Heat the mixture till it turns warm. Once the mixture has turned warm, reduce the heat to low and let it simmer.

As the milk mixture is getting warmed, take another saucepan. Add the water to it and bring it to a boil.

As the water is getting boiled, take a medium sized bowl. Add the egg yolks, whole eggs, remaining granulated sugar, cinnamon, vanilla and nutmeg to it and whisk well. Ensure that all the ingredients are mixed well. Now, add the pumpkin to the bowl and mix well. Now, add the pumpkin mixture to the milk mixture and combine well. Ensure that there are no lumps. Once the ingredients have combined well, divide the filling equally among the 8 ramekins.

Now, place the baking pan in the oven. Pour the hot water into the pan. Ensure that the water reaches at least halfway till the sides of the ramekins. Now, bake the flans for around 35 to 40 minutes. This should be sufficient time for the flans to get baked and set. At the end of 40 minutes, remove the ramekins from the oven and allow the flans to cool completely.

Take a dessert plate and invert it over one ramekin. Now, carefully lift the ramekin and invert it. The flan should slide out onto the plate, with the syrup oozing out. Use dessert plans to invert the remaining 7 ramekins in a similar fashion.

Serve the flans immediately.

Chapter 8:
Sample Diet Plans

Often, we tend to stray away from our diets due to the lack of solid planning. Planning ahead is very important to stay on track. When you plan your meals ahead, you can make sure that your pantry is well stocked with the requisite ingredients. Often, an empty pantry is what it takes to break your resolve to diet, especially if you are an amateur dieter. Similarly, when you have planned your meals in advance, you will seldom feel the itch to go and eat out. In this chapter, I have given a sample diet plan for two weeks. This should help you in kick starting this diet.

Week 1:

Day	Breakfast	Lunch	Snack	Dinner
Monday	Fluffy pancakes	Chickpea salad	Crackers and dip	Chicken kabobs
Tuesday	Yogurt granola parfait	Vegetable pot pie	Chickpea spread	Tomato and Mozzarella sandwich
Wednesday	Goat cheese and chive frittata	Turkey and artichoke sandwich	Lima bean spread	Mediterranean grilled sea bass
Thursd	Oatmeal	Leftover grilled sea	Vegetables and	Frittata and

ay	with raisins	bass from the night before	sweet sour cream dip	Baklava
Friday	Creamy and crunchy yogurt	Vegetarian Pita sandwich with Greek cucumber yogurt	Crackers with sour and sweet creamy spread	Mediterranean sweet and sour chicken
Saturday	Peanut butter with bagel and chocolate milk	Thin crust cheese pizza and green salad	Pineapple smoothie	Lamb souvlaki
Sunday	Pita with raisins and ricotta spread	Lamb chops with couscous	Raspberry banana yogurt smoothie	Basil shrimp summer salad

Week 2:

Day	Breakfast	Lunch	Snack	Dinner
Monday	Pancakes with creamy ricotta	Corn, tomato salsa and black bean salad	Nutty yogurt	Grilled chicken with Greek salad
Tuesday	Scrambled eggs and wheat toast	Veggie burger with potatoes	Raisin bran, yogurt and pecans	Tomato couscous with asparagus and crumbled ground beef
Wednesday	Granola bar	Grilled basil chicken with pasta	Flavored hummus and root vegetables	Grilled snapper
Thursday	Cereal with cherries and berries	Tuna pasta	Milk and peanut butter crackers	Chicken piccata with green salad
Friday	Kale smoothie	French toast with fruit salad	Chives spread with vegetables and sour	Spinach feta flatbread

			cream	
Saturday	Omelet with olives and vegetables	Whole grain sandwich with fresh vegetables and cheese	Apple and peanut butter	Scallops and orzo
Sunday	Blueberry and ricotta cheese mixture	Stuffed sardines	Roasted eggplant with feta dip	Mediterranean lasagna

The abovementioned diet charts will give you a sense of how this diet works and will help you design your meal plan. Ensure that you include as much variety as possible; not only to tap on the different nutrients but also to keep you excited to follow the diet. As you can see from the sample diet plans, there is at least one new recipe for the day. These small things can help you stay motivated and follow this diet without any deviations.

Conclusion

The Mediterranean Diet is rightly regarded as one of the healthiest eating plans in the world. It relies on fresh ingredients, simply cooked from scratch to bring out the true flavors of the food. The food plan includes little or no processed foods, but there are lots of fruits, vegetables and whole grains included, as well as healthy, low fat protein sources such as poultry and fish.

It's a healthy lifetime eating plan, which anyone can follow, and all the foods are readily available, wherever in the world you happen to live.